BEGINNING
T'ai Chi

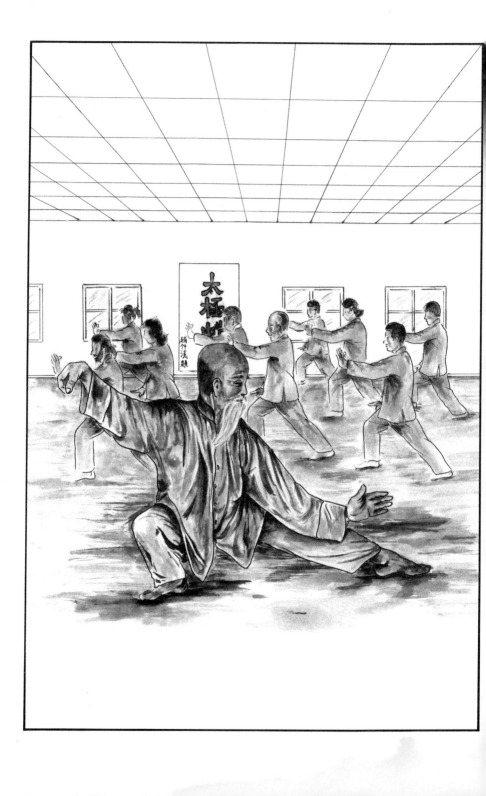

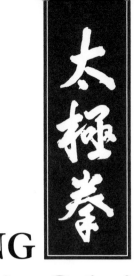

BEGINNING
T'ai Chi

Tri Thong Dang

CHARLES E. TUTTLE COMPANY
Rutland, Vermont & Tokyo, Japan

I very much appreciate the advice of my friend and editorial consultant Dr. Jonathan Pearce in the preparation of this book.

Disclaimer
Please note that the author and publisher of this instructional book are NOT RESPONSIBLE in any manner whatsoever for any injury that may result from practicing the techniques and/or following the instructions given within. Since the physical activities described herein may be too strenuous in nature for some readers to engage in safely, *it is essential that a physician be consulted prior to training.*

Published by the Charles E. Tuttle Company, Inc.
of Rutland, Vermont & Tokyo, Japan
with editorial offices at
2-6 Suido 1-chome, Bunkyo-ku, Tokyo 112

© 1994 by Tri Thong Dang

First edition, 1994

LCC Card No. 94-60562
ISBN 0-8048-2001-5

Printed in Singapore

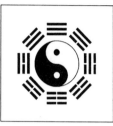 # Table of Contents

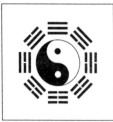 # Acknowledgments

I have been privileged to study the martial arts from my youth with many fine teachers, some of them internationally celebrated, others almost unknown but equally elegant in their simplicity, integrity, and devotion to their arts.

I am eternally bound in love and gratitude to the late Grand Master Chiu Chuk-Kai, the eighth-generation master of the Chinese T'ai-Mantis system.

He is gone from this world after more than ninety amazingly productive years, but his benevolent spirit lives on in teachings that have blessed and benefited thousands throughout the world.

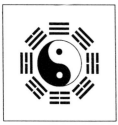 # An Introduction to the World of T'ai Chi

T'ai Chi, once an exercise practiced by only a handful of devoted disciples in China, has now become an internationally recognized and practiced art form. The international popularity of T'ai Chi has prompted me to create a text for beginners that would help familiarize them with this holistic art before beginning more formal instruction.

In the following section, I will present the information that one should know before beginning the practice of T'ai Chi. I will begin by describing the reasons why one should study T'ai Chi and illustrating the many benefits of its regular practice. Next I will briefly describe the history of T'ai Chi and why I chose to present the "Simplified T'ai Chi Form" in this book. Lastly, before beginning description of the form, I will describe how to best make use of this book as an aid in studying T'ai Chi.

Why T'ai Chi?

Perhaps you have begun this book because you have heard something about T'ai Chi and believe that reading this manual and practicing its exercises will help you become more healthful, flexible, and freer in movement and mind. Congratulations! You have made the right choice!

The graceful and lithesome movements of T'ai Chi recently have attracted worldwide attention, not only by the sports and recreation community but also by the medical profession and business persons. This is because T'ai Chi is both medicinal and practical in its effects. Whether you are seeking an exercise regimen, a path to better health, or simply a way to relax and find your "center," T'ai Chi fits the need. The movements of T'ai Chi are forms of kung fu, but the T'ai Chi forms are very different from the more combative forms of kung fu in their execution. Whereas kung fu techniques are usually swift and sometimes sharply defined, the T'ai Chi movements are part of a routine that when well executed may appear almost dreamlike in its flowing smoothness.

A Glimpse into the History of T'ai Chi

Although no official records have been found to document the origin of T'ai Chi, according to Chinese legends a man named Zhang San Feng founded the art almost eight hundred years ago. Most of our available information about the origins of T'ai Chi has been passed on orally from generation to generation, and errors and exaggerations have of course crept into the many versions.

The most interesting tale is a product of the Song* dynasty (960–1279). According to this story, Zhang one day came upon a fight between a magpie and a snake. Zhang was wonder-struck at the constant repositioning of the two creatures who shifted effortlessly from attack to defense and back again, finally breaking off, as if by mutual agreement, and going their separate ways.

For days Zhang marveled at the clinging fluidity of those movements and the wonderful appropriateness of their ever-changing attitudes. Suddenly enlightened, he saw a previously unidentified source of strength within the human body. Zhang recognized that the quality present in the martial dance of the snake and the magpie was nothing more than *softness*. Zhang saw that softness, this mysterious and powerful element, could be developed in human beings. He decided to find out how to do so. To prove that softness overcomes hardness in the fighting arts, Zhang withdrew from the world for several years to think and to test his hypothesis. He experimented in various ways until finally he achieved success.

Today Zhang's outstanding principles and method of training have been handed down as T'ai Chi Ch'uan together with its offspring Xing-yi Quan (sometimes rendered "Hsing-i Ch'uan") and Ba-gua Zhang (Pa-kua Chang). To differentiate Shaolin

* Note that other than for the term "T'ai Chi Ch'uan," which has become standard English usage, I have used the pinyin spelling for Chinese words and names. The pinyin rendering of T'ai Chi Ch'uan is Tai Ji Quan.

martial arts and other systems, masters down through the ages have classified T'ai Chi Ch'uan, Xing-yi Quan, and Ba-gua Zhang as "soft fist" schools distinct from the earlier-mentioned "hard fist" kung fu schools.

Ingeniously incorporating techniques and attitudes from Shaolin temple boxing and Daoist breathing, Zhang succeeded in creating a wondrous style that differed from all the other systems of martial arts in his time. Today Zhang's principles and method of training have been handed down as T'ai Chi.

Why This Form for the Beginner?

Conventional forms of T'ai Chi consist of eighty or more movements. These forms take a considerable amount of time to learn and perform. Many people today find it difficult to devote the time necessary to learn such lengthy routines. They exhaust their patience trying and give up. Many people are thus lost to the art.

As the correct execution of a few movements is more important than running through a lengthy routine sloppily, China's Physical Culture and Sports Commission created a shorter course called "Simplified T'ai Chi" based on the contemporary Yang Style, which traces its origins back to Master Zhang. The course presented here is that revised form. You may consider it a springboard to advanced forms, but it is also legitimate in itself.

The Basic Movements

Thirteen techniques in 24 forms comprise the basics. The first five address whole-body technique, while the remaining eight refer to movements of the hands and arms. The names attached to the forms are "classic" and relate to kung fu technique.

About Learning from a Book

It will take some practice just to orient your mind and body to the written directions for the movements. At first the instructions may seem like the printed directions that accompany some complex toys. Initially you may experience some irritation and frustration as you try to follow the illustrations and written directions so as to perform the movements "simultaneously."

Keep at it, reading the written instructions and examining the illustrations, and after a few repetitions, you will see the relationship between the text and the images. This will allow you to discover the natural flow of the movements. You may even begin to anticipate the next movement. Eventually you will reach the point at which you will have internalized the movements and are not at all conscious of which form you are manifesting, for one form will follow the other seamlessly, and you will do the entire set of 24 forms without "thinking" at all. The full cycle should take about five to six minutes to complete.

Don't worry if even after some practice your version of T'ai Chi is still idiosyncratic, and that you may not be doing everything exactly as Zhang did it! This manual is designed to acquaint you with the basic movements and provide you with the rudiments of the art, not to enable you to be an instant master. To attain the utmost satisfaction and competence in this or any other art, you will need to study with a "live" teacher. However, what you learn from this manual will give you a terrific head start, and you will be able to perform meaningful, healthful practice before you begin more formal study.

Some general principles before you begin:

- As you learn the 24 forms, strive to execute those you have learned all at the same speed as if they were one flowing form.
- Be neither tense nor limp. You are to be focused but relaxed in movement.
- Your head turns with your eyes following the leading hand.
- Any shift of weight should be flowing, not lurching.
- When following the directions *imagine yourself standing on the center of a clock face and move to the hours of the clock:* You begin by looking straight ahead to twelve o'clock, nine o'clock is 90 degrees to your left, six o'clock is directly behind you, and so on. You turn your body frequently during the 24 forms and you move about the room, always trying to maintain your orientation to your "clock."
- Notice that in the drawings the direction of the right hand and foot is indicated by a solid line, whereas a dotted line shows the direction of left hand and foot movement.
- You may perform these forms in any garb that you find comfortable. Tennis shoes are often the choice for outdoor wear; indoors, bare feet are appropriate.

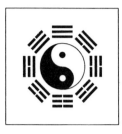

The Simplified
T'ai Chi Form

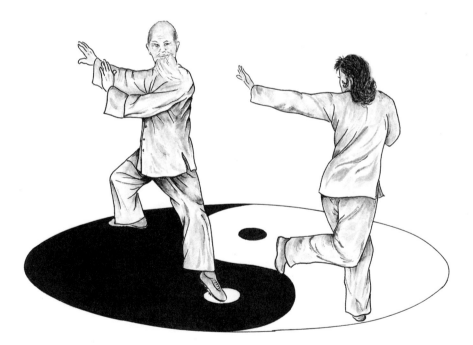

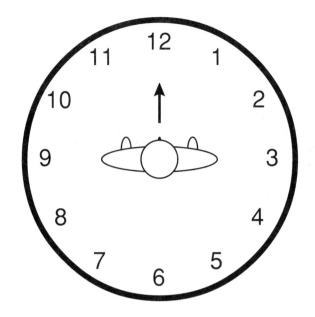

Imagine standing in the center of a clock facing twelve o'clock.

FORM ONE

Commencing

1. Stand naturally with the feet together, arms at the sides, facing twelve o'clock (Fig. 1).

2. Shift the weight slightly to the right foot. With the left foot take a half step to the left so that the feet are a shoulder's width apart (Figs. 2, 3).

3. Palms facing downward, slowly raise both arms forward to shoulder level. Then lower the arms with the palms pressing down gently while bending the knees 50–60 degrees (Figs. 4–6).

Note: The whole body should be relaxed, the back straight, and buttocks "tucked in," chin drawn slightly inward with the eyes straight forward.

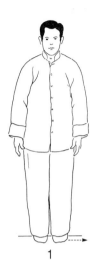

1

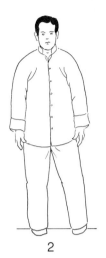

2

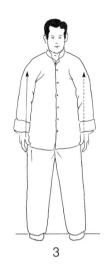

3

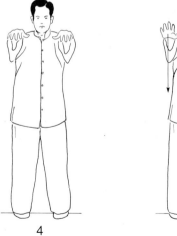

4

5

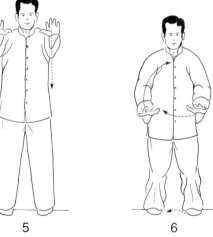

6

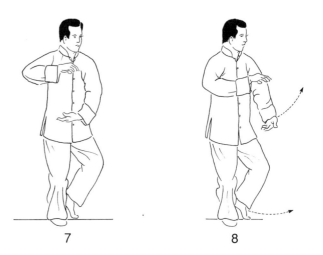

7   8

FORM TWO

Part the Horse's Mane (Both Sides)

1. Shift the weight to the right leg while turning at the waist slightly to the right (to one o'clock), and move the left foot close to the right foot with the toes on the floor. At the same time, move both hands to the left, raising the right arm smoothly to shoulder level while moving the left arm under the right. The palms face each other, as if holding a large ball. Look at the right hand (toward nine o'clock) (Figs. 7, 8).

2. Step with the left foot so that the body faces eight o'clock. Place the left heel on the floor first, then shift 70 percent of the weight forward. While doing this, push the back of the left hand forward at eye level while pressing the right hand down obliquely to the side of the right hip with the palm facing downward. Look straight forward (now nine o'clock). You are now in what is known as the "Bow stance" (Figs. 9, 10). You would not be able to hold a bow or shoot arrows in this position, but your posture is reminiscent of that of an archer.

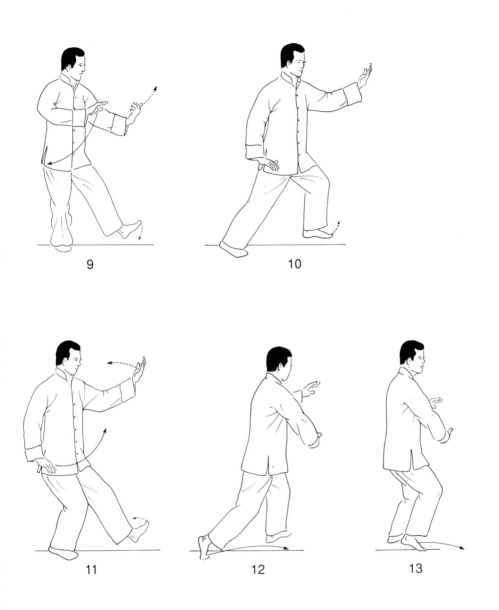

9

10

11

12

13

3. Shift the weight to the right foot, turning the left foot slightly outward (to the left). Shift the full weight back to the left foot and draw the right foot forward until it is next to the left foot with the toes on the floor. Simultaneously move both hands to the left as if holding a ball on the left side of the body (Figs. 11–13).

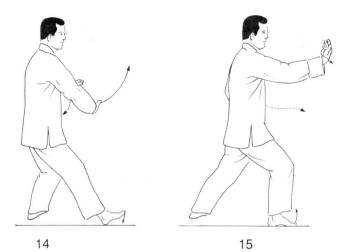

14   15

4. Turn the body to the right and take a step forward (to 10:30), placing the right heel on the floor first, and then shift 70 percent of the weight forward into the Bow stance. Simultaneously raise the right hand to eye level with the palm toward the face and eyes following the right palm. Press the left hand down obliquely to the side of the left hip (Figs. 14, 15).

5. Shift the weight to the left foot, turning the right foot slightly outward (to the right). Shift the full weight back to the right foot and draw the left foot forward until it is next to the right foot with the toes on the floor. Simultaneously move both hands to the right as if holding a ball on the right side of the body. Your eyes and head follow the right hand (Figs. 16, 17).

6. Turn the body to the left and take a step forward (toward eight o'clock), placing the left heel on the floor first, then shifting 70 percent of the weight forward into the Bow stance. At the same time, push the left hand forward at eye level, palm toward you, while pressing the right hand down obliquely to the side of the right hip. You look straight forward (at nine o'clock) (Figs. 18, 19).

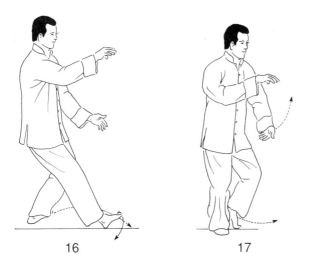

16   17

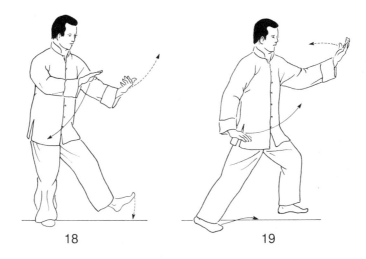

18   19

Note: During the execution of Form Two, you should keep the upper body upright but not tense, with the shoulders relaxed. In the Bow stance, the knee of the front leg should be in vertical alignment with the front elbow and toe. While you are moving through the form, try to keep your body moving at the same level rather than bobbing up and down. Try to synchronize the movement of your feet and hands so that they conclude the form at the same time.

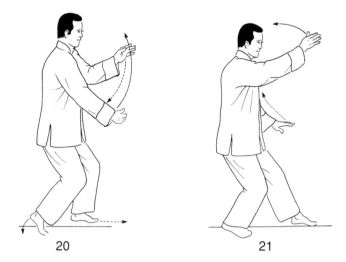

20   21

FORM THREE

White Crane Spreads Its Wings

1. From the Bow stance that ends Form Two, shift the full weight to the front (left) leg. Draw the right leg a half step forward and place it behind the left foot. Now shift the weight back to the right leg in the "Sit Back" position. Extend the left leg gently forward into what is known as the "Empty stance."

2. Turn the body slightly to the right, draw the left hand down in front of the face, and move the right hand forward, palm up, as if both hands were holding a ball, and continue the movement of both arms outward into the "White Crane Spreads Its Wings" position. You are now looking forward (at nine o'clock) (Figs. 20, 21).

Note: At the conclusion of this form, the right hand stops in front of and slightly above the right temple with the palm facing inward, and the left hand stops level with the left hip with the palm facing downward. Keep the upper body upright. Remember that when you read "stop," the word is used only to give you a marker for the technical conclusion of the form. You actually keep on moving through to the next form, relaxed, focused, and fluid!

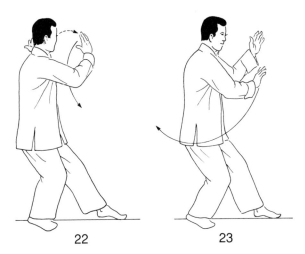

22   23

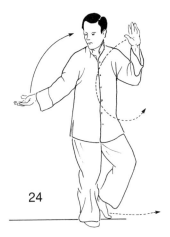

24

FORM FOUR

Brush Knee (Both Sides)

1. From the White Crane Spreads Its Wings position, turn slightly to the left (to eight o'clock). The right arm moves down in front of the face while the left arm circles up, outward, and then across the face. Both arms continue moving to the right. Simultaneously draw the left foot next to the right foot with the toes on the floor. Keep the weight of the body on the right leg with the knee bent 50–60 degrees. You are looking at the right hand (toward nine o'clock) (Figs. 22–24).

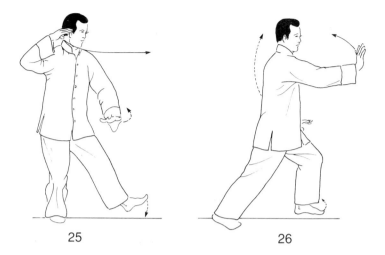

25 26

2. Turn the body to the left and take a step forward with the left leg (toward eight o'clock), placing the heel on the floor first. Circle the left hand downward so that it passes in front of the abdomen and ends at the side of the left hip. At the same time, bend the right arm toward the right ear with the palm facing obliquely forward, and push forward at shoulder level while shifting the body forward, ending in the Bow stance. Look at the right hand (at nine o'clock) (Figs. 25, 26).

3. Shift the weight back to the right foot in the Sit Back position, turning the left toes outward (to the left), and shift the full weight back to the left foot. Draw the right foot to the left foot with the toes on the floor. At the same time, bend the right arm and move the right hand before the face. Circle the left arm outward and back, and then to the front across the face (Figs. 27–29).

Note: "Sit Back" is a figurative term; one does not sit at all!

4. Turn the body to the right, take a step forward with the right leg (to ten o'clock), placing the heel on the floor first. Circle the

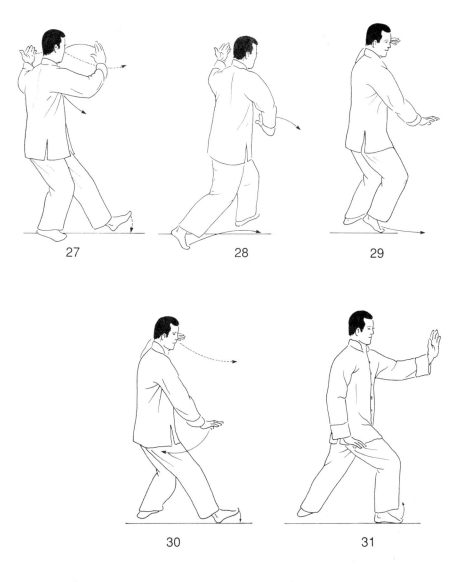

27   28   29

30   31

right hand downward, passing it in front of the abdomen and ending by the side of the right hip. At the same time, bend the left hand toward the left ear with the palm facing obliquely forward and push forward at shoulder level while shifting the body forward, ending in the Bow stance. Look toward nine o'clock (Figs. 30, 31).

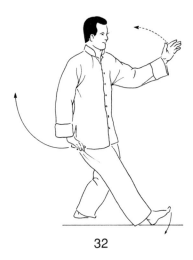

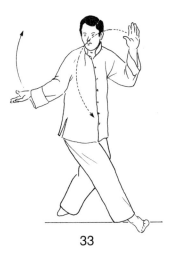

32 33

5. Shift the weight back to the left leg in the Sit Back position, turning the right toes outward (to the right). Shift the full weight forward to the right foot and draw the left foot close to the right foot with the toes on the floor. Simultaneously move the left hand before the face while circling the right hand outward and back, then toward the right ear (Figs. 32–35).

6. Turn the body to the left, and take a step forward with the left leg (toward eight o'clock) by placing the heel on the floor first. Circle the left hand downward, passing it in front of the abdomen and ending on the left side of the left hip. Simultaneously push with the right hand, palm forward, and shift the body forward, ending in the Bow stance. Look at the right hand (toward nine o'clock) (Figs. 36, 37).

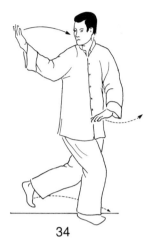

34

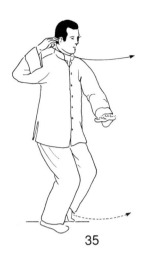

35

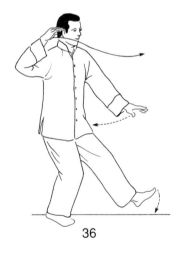

36

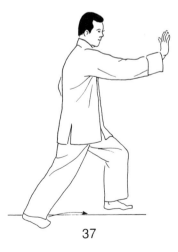

37

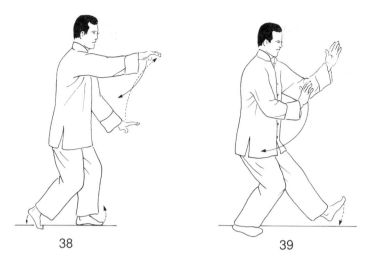

38   39

Hands Strum the Lute

1. Shift the weight to the front leg, and draw the right foot a half step forward and place it behind the left foot. Shift the weight back to the right foot to form the Sit Back position. Extend the left foot forward, ending in the Empty stance with the left toes up. Simultaneously turn the body slightly to the right, raise the left hand forward until it is level with the nose, and move the right hand horizontally to the inside of the left elbow. Look at the left hand (toward nine o'clock) (Figs. 38, 39).

Note: The shifting of the body should be synchronized with the movement of the hands so that both are completed at the same time. As you move, keep the body at the same level. It may be tempting to bob up and down, but accomplished Lute-strummers do not do so!

Step Back and Roll Arms (Both Sides)

1. Turn the body to the right and move the right hand downward in a semicircle to shoulder level with the palm up while extending

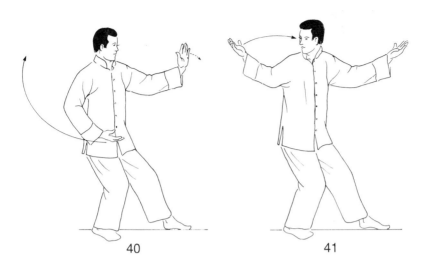

40   41

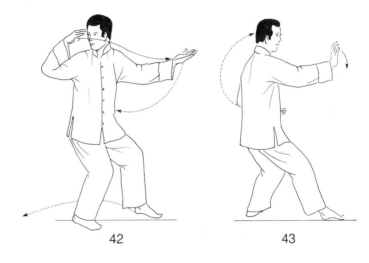

42   43

the left arm with the palm up. The left foot flattens to the floor (Figs. 40, 41).

2. Bring the right hand toward the right ear and turn the body to the left. Push the right hand forward and bring the left hand beside the waist with the palm up. At the same time, raise the left foot and step back into the Empty stance with the body weight on the left foot. Look at the right hand (toward nine o'clock) (Figs. 42, 43).

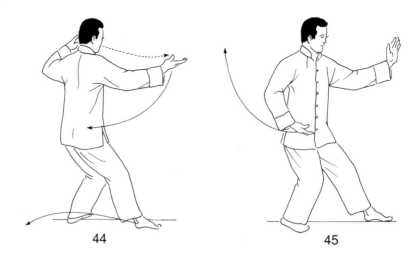

44   45

3. Bring the left hand toward the left ear and turn the body to the right. Simultaneously push the left hand forward and bring the right hand back beside the waist with the palm up. At the same time, raise the right foot and step back into the Empty stance with the body weight on the right foot. Look at the left hand (toward nine o'clock) (Figs. 44, 45).

4. Bring the right hand toward the right ear and turn the body to the left. Push the right hand forward and bring the left hand back beside the waist with the palm up. At the same time, raise the left foot and step back into the Empty stance with the body weight on the left foot. Look at the right hand (toward nine o'clock) (Figs. 46–48).

5. Circle the left hand back toward the left ear and turn the body to the right. Simultaneously push the left hand forward and bring the right hand back beside the waist with the palm up. With the hands in motion, raise the right foot and step back in the Empty stance with the body weight on the right foot. Look at the left hand (toward nine o'clock) (Figs. 49, 50).

Note: When stepping backward, always place the toes on the floor first, then slowly shift the full weight to that foot.

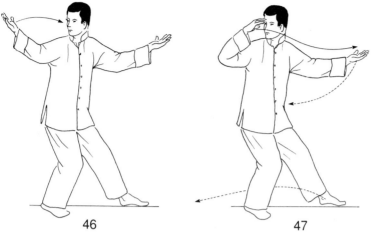

46

47

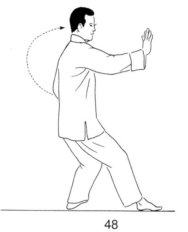

48

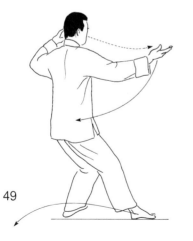

49

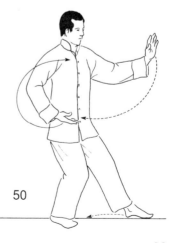

50

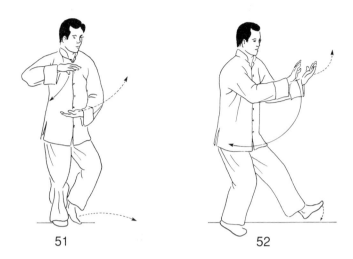

51   52

Grasp the Bird's Tail (Left Side)

1. At the end of Form Six, turn the body to the right, move the left hand downward, and bring up the right hand in a circular motion. The right hand is above the left with the palms facing, as if holding a ball. Simultaneously draw the left foot beside the right with the toes on the floor. Look at the right hand (toward eleven o'clock) (Fig. 51).

2. Turn the body to the left (to nine o'clock) and take a step to the left with the left leg, placing the heel on the floor first. Shift 70 percent of the weight forward into the Bow stance. Push the back of the left hand forward at eye level. Your eyes follow the left hand while the right hand presses down obliquely to the side of the right hip with the palm down and the fingers pointing forward. Look at the left hand (toward nine o'clock) (Figs. 52, 53).

3. Extend the right arm forward with the palm up and simultaneously turn the left palm down. Bring both arms first downward and then, in an arc, raise them backward to the right at shoulder level (toward one o'clock). During that movement, shift your weight to the right foot (Figs. 54–56). Turn the body back to the left

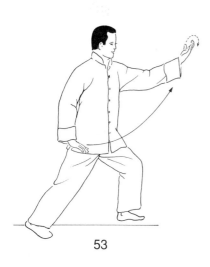

53

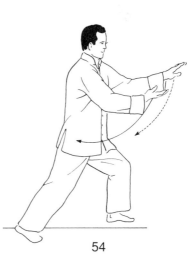

54

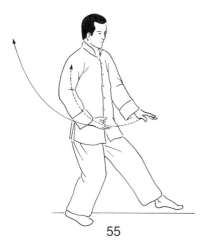

55

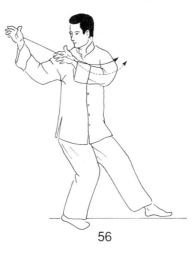

56

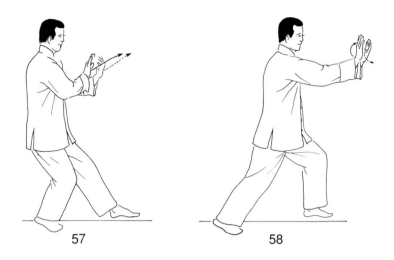

57   58

(to nine o'clock), bring the right hand close to the left wrist, and press both hands forward with the palms facing each other in front of the chest. Shift the weight to the left leg into the Bow stance. Look straight forward (now at nine o'clock) (Figs. 57, 58).

4. As both hands press forward, at the last second turn both palms down with the right crossing over left, then separate the hands until they are a shoulder width apart. Shift the weight back to the right foot into the Sit Back position with the left toes up. While shifting the weight back, pull both arms back toward the chest and down to the waist. Look straight forward (Figs. 59–62).

5. Move the weight forward into the Bow stance while pushing both hands forward and upward to shoulder level. Continue looking straight forward (toward nine o'clock) (Fig. 63).

Note: While pushing the hands forward, keep the upper body straight and the shoulders relaxed. The movement of the arms and the shifting of the weight must end simultaneously.

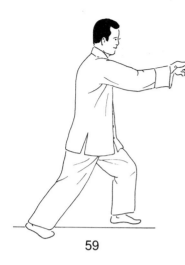

59

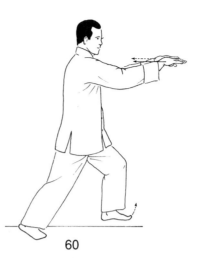

60

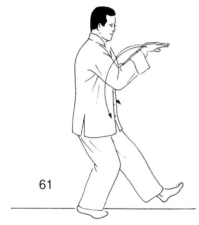

61

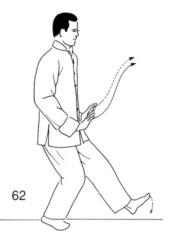

62

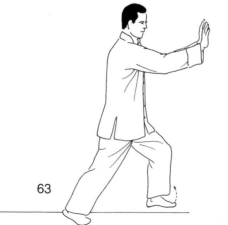

63

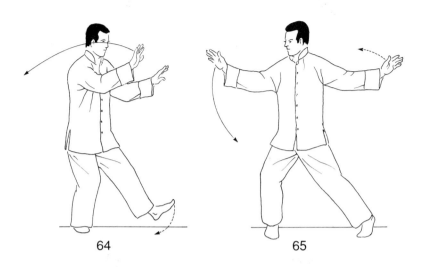

64   65

Grasp the Bird's Tail (Right Side)

1. Shift the weight back to the right foot and pivot inward on the right heel. Move the right arm to the right, curve it down, and pass the abdomen with the palm up. Bring the left arm to the right until both palms face each other, as if holding a ball. Simultaneously shift the weight back to the left leg, and draw the right foot close to the left foot. Look at the left hand (Figs. 64–67).

2. Turn the body to the right (toward three o'clock) and take a step to the right with the right leg (to four o'clock), placing the heel on the floor first. Shift 70 percent of the weight forward into the Bow stance. At the same time, push the back of the right hand forward at eye level while the left hand presses down obliquely to the side of the left hip with the palm down and fingers pointing forward. Look at the right hand (toward three o'clock) (Figs. 68, 69).

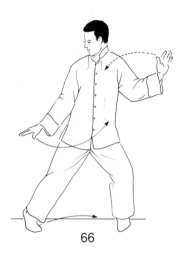

66

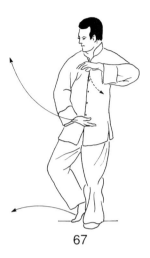

67

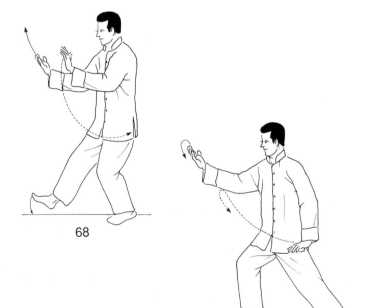

68

69

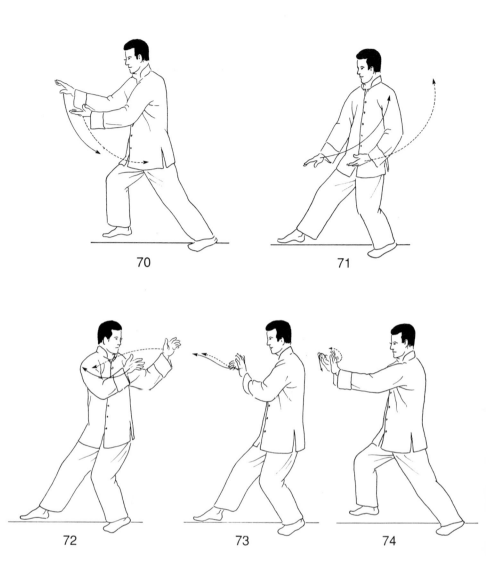

70

71

72

73

74

3. Extend the left arm with the palm up and turn the right palm down while shifting the weight back to the left leg. Pull both arms downward and raise them across the body in an arc to the left at shoulder level (toward eleven o'clock). Turn the body back to the right, bringing the left hand close to the right wrist, and pressing both hands forward with the palms facing each other in front of the chest. Simultaneously shift the weight to the right leg into the Bow stance. Look straight forward at the hands (toward three o'clock) (Figs. 70–74).

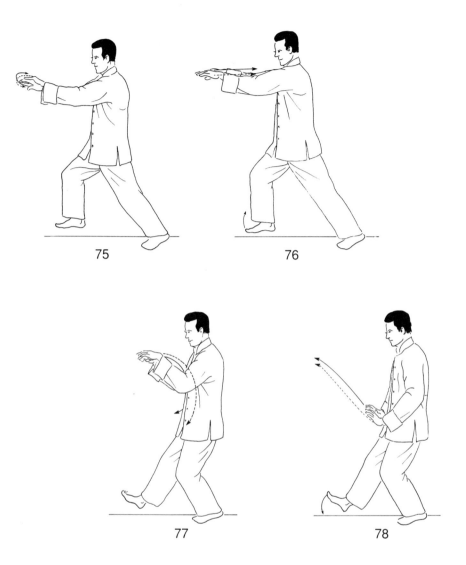

75

76

77

78

4. As both hands press forward, at the last second turn both palms down, the left crossing over right, then separate the hands until they are a shoulder width apart. Shift the weight back to the left leg in the Sit Back position with the right toes up. At the same time, pull back both hands, palms down, toward the chest and down to the waist. Look straight forward (toward three o'clock) (Figs. 75–78).

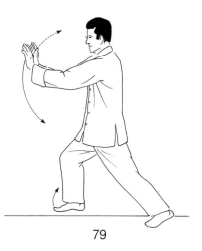

79

5. Move the weight forward into the Bow stance while pushing both hands forward, and upward, to shoulder level. Look straight forward (toward three o'clock) (Fig. 79).

Note: While pushing the hands forward, keep the upper body straight and the shoulders relaxed. The movement of the arms and the shifting of the weight end at the same time. Notice that Form Eight is the mirror image of Form Seven!

FORM NINE

Single Whip

1. Shift the weight to the left into the Sit Back position, then pivot to the left on the right heel with the toes turning inward. Turn the body to the left while the left hand passes in front of the face and the right hand passes in front of the abdomen and continues upward in a circular motion to the left at shoulder level. Look at the left hand (toward ten o'clock) (Figs. 80, 81).

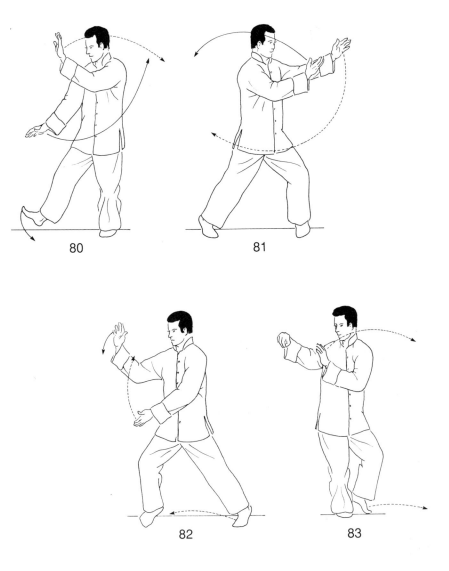

80   81

82   83

2. Shift the weight back to the right leg while the right palm passes in front of the face, ending in a Hook hand. Simultaneously the left hand moves downward, passing the abdomen, and then upward with the palm ending inside the right elbow. Pull the left foot back close to the right foot with the toes on the floor. Look at the Hook hand (toward one o'clock) (Figs. 82, 83).

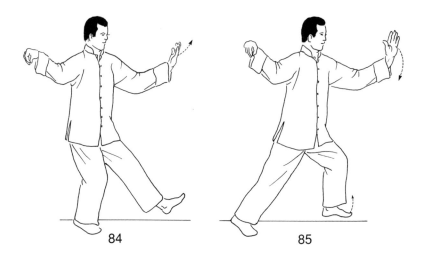

84　　　　　　　　　85

3. Turn the body to the left (to nine o'clock), and take a step forward with the left leg (toward eight o'clock), placing the heel on the floor. Simultaneously move the left arm to the left while turning the palm outward. Shift the weight to the left foot in the Bow stance. Look at the left hand (toward nine o'clock) (Figs. 84, 85).

Note: Keep the upper body straight but not tense while shifting the weight. Shoulders and waist are always relaxed. At the end of the movement both arms are slightly bent and the left elbow is in line with and above the left knee.

FORM TEN

Wave Hands Like Clouds (Left Side)

1. From Form Nine, shift the weight to the right leg. At the same time, turn the body to the right and pivot on the left heel until the left foot is pointed forward. Circle the left arm down and then upward to the right at shoulder level. The left palm turns up and the right hand (the Hook hand) is open with the palm down. Look at the left hand (toward two o'clock) (Figs. 86, 87).

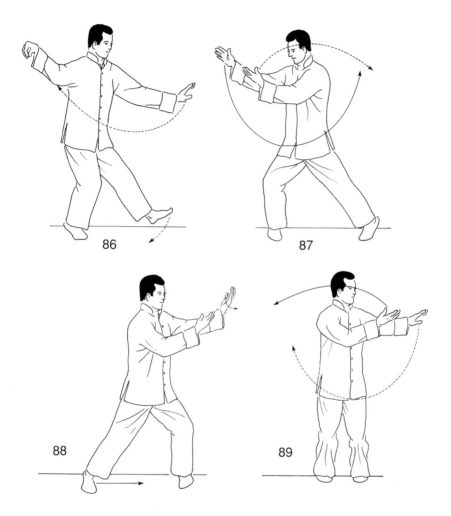

2. Turn the body to the left and shift the weight to the left leg. Move the left hand to the left in front of the face and the right hand downward, passing the abdomen, and then upward, until both hands are level with the left shoulder. Simultaneously draw the right foot to the left foot until both feet are parallel and about a foot apart. Look at the left hand (toward nine o'clock) (Figs. 88, 89).

Note: While moving, maintain the body height. Don't bob and weave! Footwork and arm movement should be coordinated in a flowing motion.

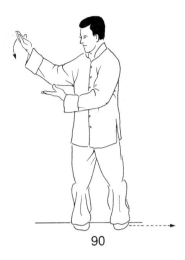

90

3. Turn the body to the right and shift the weight to the right leg. At the same time, circle the right arm to the right, passing it in front of the face, and circle the left arm downward, passing it in front of the abdomen and then upward and level with the right shoulder (Fig. 90).

4. Take a step sideways with the left leg and shift the weight to it. At the same time, circle the left hand, passing it in front of the face and moving the right hand downward in a circular motion until both hands are level with the right shoulder. Draw the right leg to the left foot until both feet are parallel and about a foot apart. Look at the left hand (toward nine o'clock) (Figs. 91–93).

5. Turn the upper body to the right and shift the weight to the right leg. At the same time, circle the right arm to the right, passing it in front of the face, and circle the left arm downward, palm down, passing the abdomen and then moving upward to shoulder level with the palm facing inward. Look at the right hand (toward three o'clock) (Fig. 94).

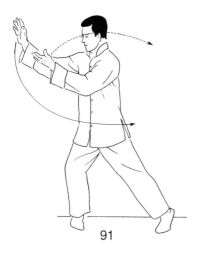

91

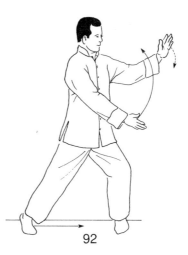

92

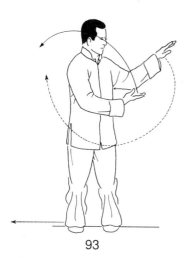

93

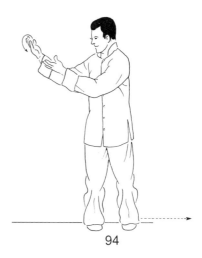

94

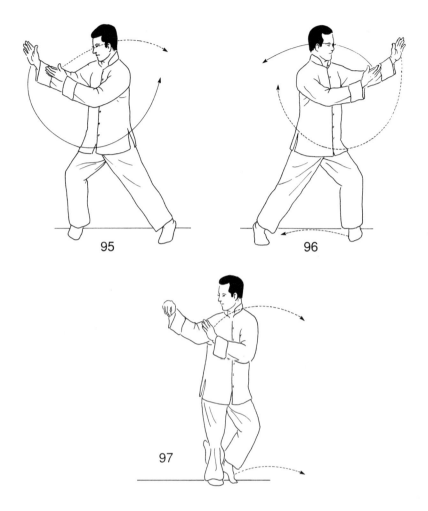

95

96

97

6. Take a step sideways with the left leg and shift the weight to the left leg. Simultaneously circle the left hand to the left, passing it in front of the face. Move the right hand downward in a curve so that it passes the abdomen and then up again so that both hands are at the level of the left shoulder (toward nine o'clock). Circle the right hand back to the right, passing it in front of the face and ending in a Hook hand on the right. At the same time, move the left hand down, passing the abdomen and ending at the inside of the right elbow. Simultaneously draw the left foot close to the right foot. Look at the right hand (Figs. 95–97).

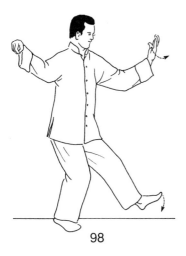

98

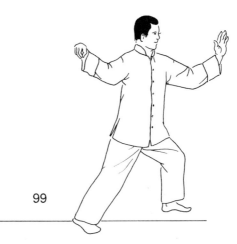

99

Single Whip

1. Move the left arm to the left, turning the palm outward (to nine o'clock). Take a step forward with the left leg (to eight o'clock), placing the heel on the floor first, and then gradually shift the weight to the left leg into the Bow stance. Look at the left palm (Figs. 98, 99).

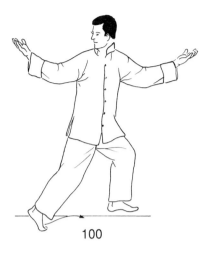

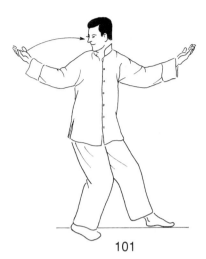

100   101

High Pat the Horse

1. From the Bow stance position, shift the weight to the front leg, draw the right foot a half step forward and place it behind the left foot. Shift the weight back to the right leg. Simultaneously open the right Hook hand and turn both palms up with the elbows slightly bent. Look at the right hand (Figs. 100, 101).

2. Turn the body to the left (to nine o'clock). Move the right hand past the right ear and push the palm forward. At the same time, draw the left arm to the left side of the hip with the palm facing upward, and gently slide the left foot forward, ending in the Empty stance. Look at the right hand (Figs. 102, 103).

Note: When shifting the weight, maintain the same height with the upper body straight and the right elbow slightly bent.

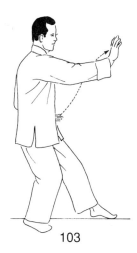

102

103

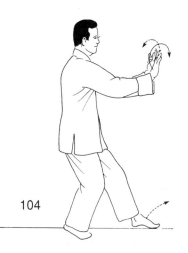

104

Kick with the Right Heel

1. Turn the upper body slightly to the right (to ten o'clock), and cross the left hand over the right wrist (Fig. 104).

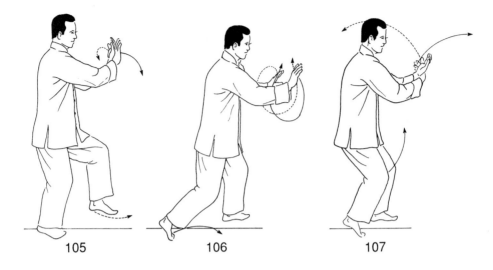

105   106   107

2. Take a step forward with the left leg (to eight o'clock) and shift the full weight to it. Separate the hands, making a small downward circle until they cross again with both palms facing inward, the left hand over the right (Figs. 105–107).

3. Without stopping, continue circling the hands, extending both arms sideways at shoulder level while bringing the right leg forward and kicking out slowly with the right heel (to ten o'clock). Look at the right hand (Figs. 108, 109).

Note: When bringing the right hand forward, the right knee is higher than the hip. While kicking with the right heel, the left leg is slightly bent. The right arm is extended over and in the direction of the right leg. The kick is executed at the same speed as the rest of the exercise.

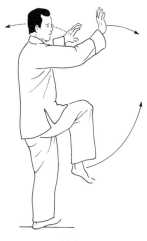

108

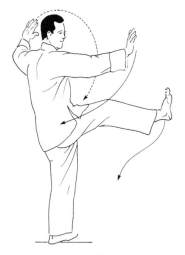

109

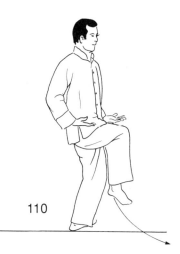

110

Strike the Opponent's Ears with Both Fists

1. After kicking, pull back the right leg, and at the same time draw both arms downward to either side of the body with the palms turning upward (Fig. 110).

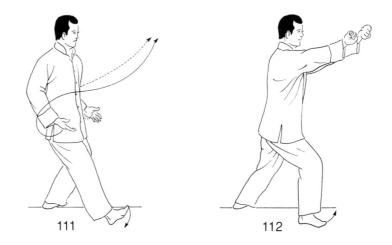

111   112

2. Take a step with the right leg (to ten o'clock), and shift the weight to it, forming the Bow stance. Simultaneously clench the hands into fists. Extend them upward from either side, ending at the level of the temple with the knuckles pointing obliquely upward about six inches apart. Look straight between the two fists (Figs. 111, 112).

Note: Keep the upper body straight, but not tense, and the arms relaxed. When extending the fists, your eyes should focus on the left fist until the movement is concluded.

FORM FIFTEEN

Turn and Kick with the Left Heel

1. Shift the weight back to the left leg. Turn the body to the left while pivoting on the right heel with the toes turning inward. Shift the weight back to the right leg and simultaneously open both hands with the palms upward. Move both arms downward and sideways. Look at the left hand (Figs. 113, 114).

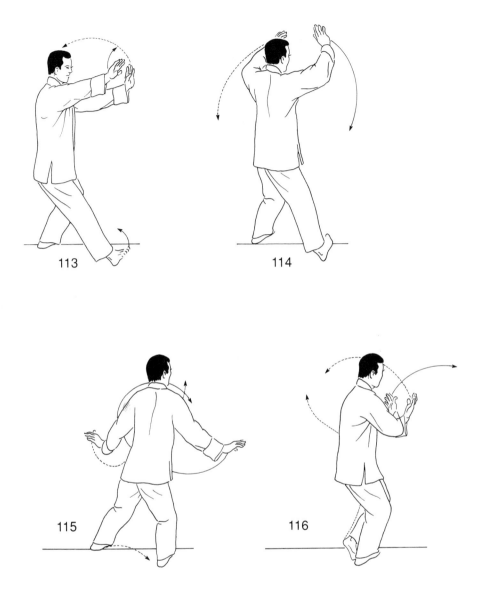

113

114

115

116

2. As soon as the weight is completely transferred to the right leg, draw the left foot to the side of the right foot with the toes on the floor. Both arms continue to move up in a circle and cross at the wrists in front of the chest with the palms facing inward, the right hand over the left. Look at the left hand (Figs. 115, 116).

3. Separate the hands, extending them sideways horizontally at shoulder level with the elbows slightly bent. At the same time, raise the left leg and kick out slowly with the left heel (to four o'clock). Look at the left hand (Fig. 117).

Note: While kicking with the left heel, the right leg is slightly bent. Foot and hand motion should be executed simultaneously. The direction of the left kick is opposite to the direction of the right kick. The left arm is extended in the direction of the left leg.

FORM SIXTEEN

Push Down and Stand on One Leg (Left Side)

1. After kicking with the left leg, pull back the leg as the right hand turns into a Hook hand and the left hand moves slowly to the inside of the right elbow. Look at the right hand (Fig. 118).

2. Turn the body to the left (to three o'clock). Crouch down slowly on the right leg and stretch the left leg sideways (to two o'clock), the toes turning inward with both feet on the floor. At the same time, move the left hand down, parallel to the body inside the left leg. Turn the palms outward. Look at the left hand (Fig. 119).

3. Pivot on the left heel, turning the toes outward and moving the body up and forward (to three o'clock). Straighten the right leg and bend the left into the Bow stance. Simultaneously, move the left hand up, palm facing right, and turn the right arm up behind and parallel to the body with a Hook hand. The fingers of the right hand are pointing backward and upward. Look at three o'clock (Fig. 120).

4. Move the body forward and up while shifting the full weight to the left leg. Simultaneously open the right hand and move it up in a circle, with the palm facing the left side, ending in front of the face at eye level. At the same time, the left hand presses down to the side of the left hip with the palm down as you raise the right knee. Look at the right hand (at three o'clock) (Figs. 121, 122).

Note: Bend the supporting leg (the left leg) slightly. The knee of the raised leg must be higher than the hip, and the foot hangs naturally.

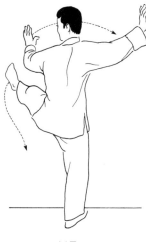

117

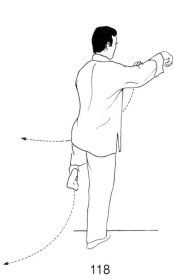

118

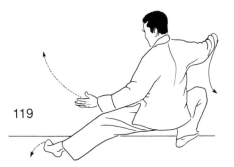

119

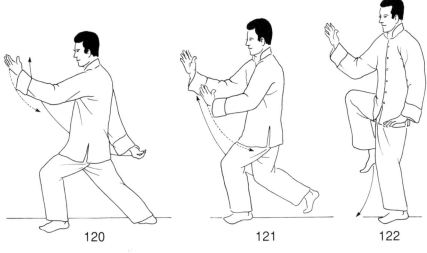

120

121

122

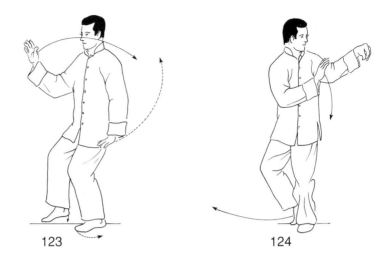

123   124

Push Down and Stand on One Leg (Right Side)

1. Turn the body slightly to the left, lower the right foot in front of the left foot, and shift the weight fully to the right leg. Turn the left foot slightly to the left by pivoting on the ball of the foot, and shift the weight back fully to the left leg. At the same time, raise the left hand to shoulder level and form a Hook hand while the right hand moves to the inside of the elbow of the left arm. Look at the left hand (toward eleven o'clock) (Figs. 123, 124).

2. Turn the body slowly back to the right, crouch down slowly on the left leg, and stretch the right leg sideways (to four o'clock) with the toes pointing inward. Both feet are flat on the floor. At the same time, move the right hand down, parallel to the body and inside the right leg. Look at the right hand (Figs. 125, 126).

3. Pivot on the right heel, turning the toes outward, and moving the body up and forward (to three o'clock). Straighten the left leg and bend the right knee into the Bow stance. At the same time, move the right hand up with the palm facing left while the left arm turns up behind and parallel to the body in a Hook hand. The fingers of the left hand are pointing backward and upward. Look at the right hand (Fig. 127).

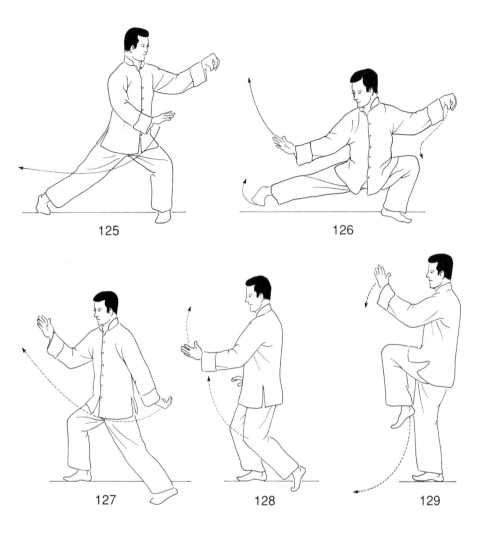

125

126

127

128

129

4. Move the body forward and up while shifting the full weight to the right leg. At the same time, open the left hand and move it up in a circle, with the palm facing the right side, ending in front of the face at eye level. Simultaneously the right hand presses down to the side of the right hip with the palm down as you raise your left knee. Look at the left hand (Figs. 128, 129).

Note: Bend the supporting leg (the right leg) slightly. The knee of the right leg must be higher than the hip, and the foot hangs naturally.

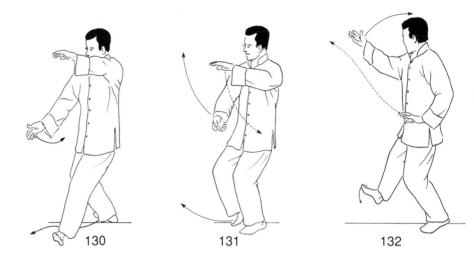

130   131   132

Work at Shuttles (Both Sides)

1. Bend the right knee, turn the body to the left (to one o'clock), and take a step forward with the left leg. The left foot crosses in front of the right and the toes turn outward. Shift the full weight to the left foot and move the right foot close to the left foot with the toes on the floor. Lower the left arm horizontally to shoulder level and move the right hand to the left until both palms face each other, as if holding a ball. Look at the left hand (Figs. 130, 131).

2. Turn the body slightly to the right and take a step forward with the right leg (to four o'clock). Place the heel on the floor first and then shift 70 percent of the weight forward into the Bow stance. At the same time, raise the right arm in front of the right forehead, with the palm turned outward while moving the left hand down in a circular motion to the left waist. Push the left arm forward up to eye level. Look at the left hand (Figs. 132, 133).

3. Shift the weight back to the left foot and turn the right toes slightly outward. Shift the weight back to the right leg while drawing the left foot close to the right foot with the toes on the floor. At the same time, lower the right arm to shoulder level and move the left arm down in front of the body until the palms face each other, as if holding a ball. Look at the right hand (Figs. 134, 135).

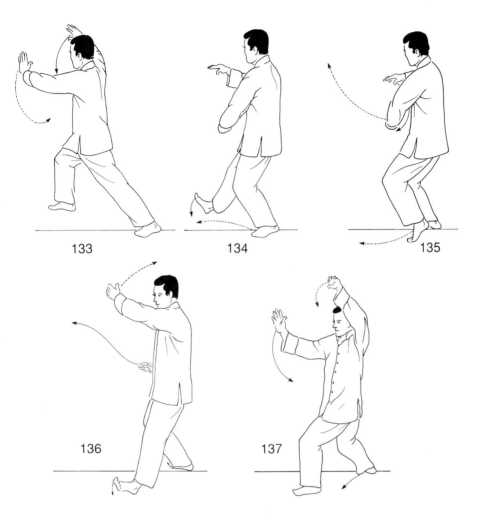

133   134   135

136   137

4. Turn the body to the left and take a step forward with the left leg (to two o'clock), placing the heel on the floor first, then shifting 70 percent of the weight forward into the Bow stance. At the same time, raise the left arm up in front of the left forehead, with the palm turning outward while moving the right hand down in a circular motion to the right waist. Push the right arm forward again up to eye level. Look at the right hand (Figs. 136, 137).

Note: While moving, maintain the same body level and keep the back straight and shoulders relaxed. Keep in mind that all 24 forms comprise one motion, accomplished at one speed.

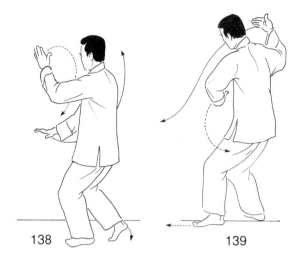
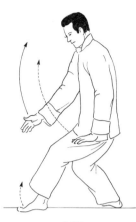

138   139   140

Needle at the Bottom of the Sea

1. Shift the weight to the left foot and take a half step forward with the right leg, placing the toes behind the left foot then shifting the full weight to the right foot. Gently extend the left foot forward into the Empty stance. Turn the body to the right (to four o'clock), and circle the right arm to the right and up to the right temple with the fingers pointing directly downward in front of the body. At the same time, the left hand moves to the right in front of the face and down to the left side of the hip with the palm down and fingers pointing forward. Look at the floor in front of your feet (toward three o'clock) (Figs. 138–140).

Note: Keep the left leg slightly bent and the upper body as upright as possible.

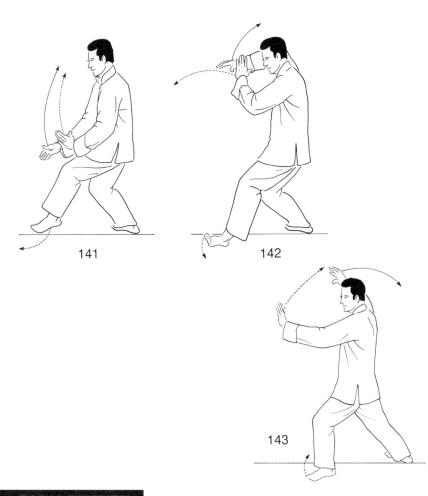

141   142

143

Flash Arm

1. Take a step forward with the left foot and shift the weight forward into the Bow stance. At the same time, raise both hands and cross them at the wrists in front of the right temple. Push the left palm forward at the level of the nose, as the right palm turns outward above the right side of the head. Look at the left hand (at two o'clock) (Figs. 141–143).

Note: During the execution of this form, keep the upper body upright and the waist relaxed. Footwork and hand motion should be synchronized to end at the same time.

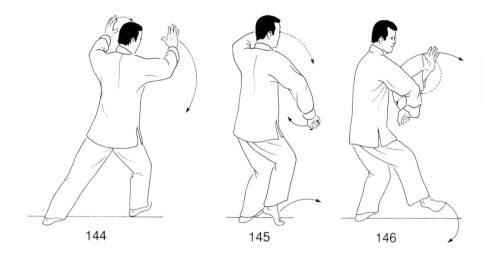

144   145   146

Turn and Deflect Downward, Parry, and Punch

1. Shift the weight to the right leg, pivoting on the left heel with the toes turning inward. Shift the full weight back to the left foot while facing six o'clock. While turning to the right, lower both arms in a circle, close the right hand into a fist, and move the left hand in front of the forehead. At the same time, pull the right foot close to the left foot (Figs. 144, 145).

2. During this turning of the body to the right, the right fist continues to move down and circles in front of the stomach and the back of the fist turns upward. The left hand moves down in front of the face and then down to the side of the left hip with the palm facing downward. Take a step forward with the right leg (toward ten o'clock). Look at the right fist (Figs. 146, 147).

3. Shift the weight to the right foot. Draw the left foot forward with the heel touching the floor first. The left hand moves up in front of the face, and the right fist moves down and rotates on the right side of the right hip. Look at the left hand (at nine o'clock) (Figs. 148, 149).

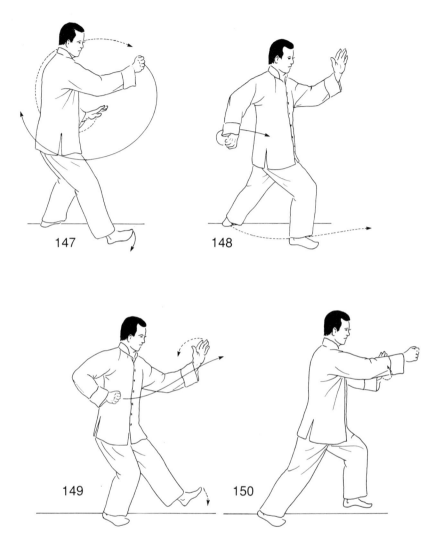

147

148

149

150

4. Shift the weight to the left foot to form the Bow stance while parrying with the left hand and striking forward with the right fist at shoulder level. Look at the right fist (at nine o'clock) (Fig. 150).

Note: When executing the punch, the shoulder should be relaxed, arm slightly bent, and fist loosely clenched. The thumb side of the fist is up. The "blow" is delivered at the same speed at which the rest of the exercise is performed.

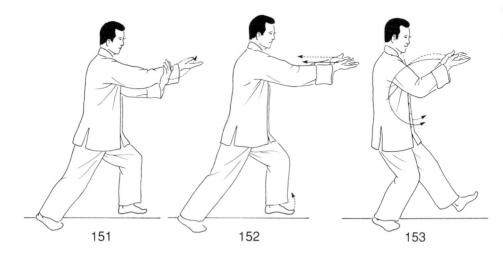

151   152   153

Apparent Close

1. Turn the left hand under the right forearm and open the right hand with both palms now facing upward. Separate the hands until they are a shoulder width apart, and pull them back toward the chest and then down to the sides of the waist. At the same time, shift the weight back to the right foot to form the Sit Back position with the left toes up. Look forward (to nine o'clock) (Figs. 151–154).

2. Shift your weight forward into the Bow stance while pushing the hands forward and upward to shoulder level. Continue looking forward (toward nine o'clock) (Fig. 155).

Note: Try always to keep the shoulders relaxed and the upper body straight but not tense. After pushing the hands forward, both hands are a shoulder width apart and the arms are slightly bent.

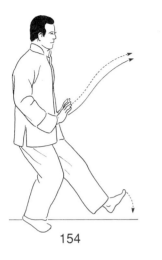

154

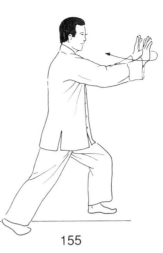

155

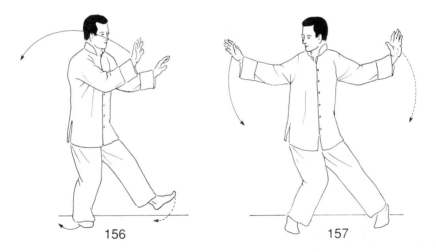

156   157

Cross Hands

1. Shift the weight back to the right leg and turn the body to the right while moving the right arm down in a circle. Simultaneously pivot on the left heel and then return the toes to the floor. The toes should be now facing forward. Look at the right hand (Figs. 156, 157).

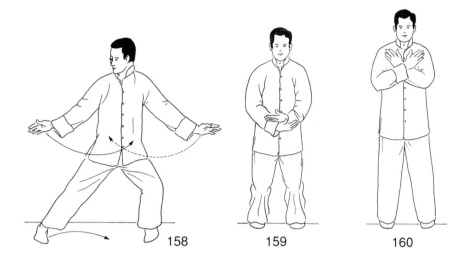

158 159 160

2. Shift the weight back to the left leg while lowering both arms until they cross with the palms facing inward. Move the arms up to the level of the chest. Simultaneously, draw the right leg toward the left foot until both feet are parallel and a shoulder width apart. Look straight forward (to twelve o'clock) (Figs. 158–160).

Note: During the shifting of the weight, try not to lean the body forward.

FORM TWENTY-FOUR

Closing Form

1. Extend both arms forward while turning the palms down. Separate the hands until they are a shoulder width apart. Lower both arms slowly to the sides of the hips. Look straight forward (to twelve o'clock) (Figs. 161–163).

2. Shift the weight to the right foot and draw the left foot toward the right foot. Continue looking straight forward (to twelve o'clock) (Figs. 164, 165).

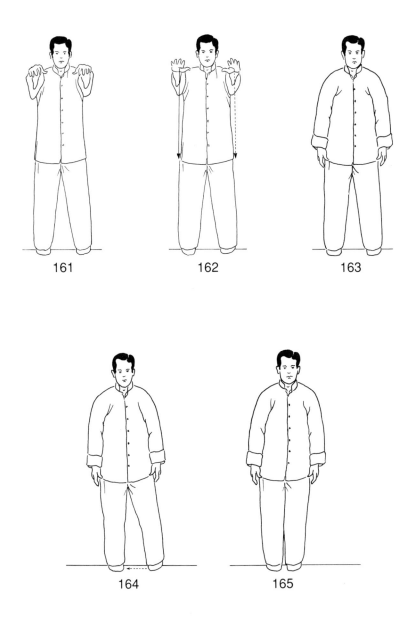

161 162 163

164 165

You have completed the cycle. You may repeat it as many times as you wish, but at least four times, always being sure to breathe naturally and regularly. Attaining speed is not a criterion in T'ai Chi, but achieving smoothness of execution is.

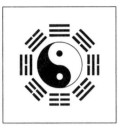 # Conclusion

As you learn the routine by repeating it numerous times and checking your movements against the illustrations in this book (observing your progress in a mirror may be helpful at first), please reflect on the following points:

- The 24 forms are to be executed seamlessly—without pause.
- The routine is performed at one speed: slow. The 24 forms can be completed in about five to six minutes. Ideally, even the kicks are performed at the same speed as the rest of the movements.
- When shifting weight from one foot to the other, the moving foot is fully placed on the ground before any weight is shifted.
- You are almost certain to "think" about what you are doing while you are learning the routine. That is natural. However, after you have learned the movements, let your body do the thinking.

After you have learned the rudiments of T'ai Chi from this manual, it will be very helpful for you to train with a teacher. After you have refined your technique with the help of the teacher for a time, you can learn to develop your own potential, something you alone must do. In so doing, your knowledge and practice of T'ai Chi will surely enrich your life.

Other Titles in the Tuttle Library of Martial Arts

AIKIDO AND THE DYNAMIC SPHERE
by Adele Westbrook and Oscar Ratti

Aikido is a Japanese method of self-defense that can be used against any form of attack and that is also a way of harmonizing all of one's vital powers into an integrated, energy-filled whole.

BEGINNING QIGONG: CHINESE SECRETS OF FITNESS *by Stephen Kuei and Stephen Comee*

A straightforward, easy-to-use text on this powerful art of self-healing. Learn the Chinese secrets of health and longevity through these easy and graceful exercises.

BEYOND THE KNOWN: THE ULTIMATE GOAL OF THE MARTIAL ARTS *by Tri Thong Dang*

A novel that illustrates one man's quest to find the way of the martial arts. A work that will make you question your motives and goals, and go beyond the dazzle of prizes and awards, beyond the repetition of techniques, and beyond the known—the ultimate goal of the arts.

BLACK BELT KARATE *by Jordan Roth*

A no-frills, no-holds-barred handbook on the fundamentals of modern karate. Over 800 techniques and exercises and more than 1,850 photographs reveal the speed and power inherent in properly taught karate.

COMPLETE TAI-CHI: THE DEFINITIVE GUIDE TO PHYSICAL AND EMOTIONAL SELF-IMPROVEMENT *by Alfred Huang*

A step-by-step guide to the practice, history, and philosophy of Wu-style Tai-chi. Including unique English translations of original Chinese texts, it is the most complete work on this holistic and spiritual art.

THE ESSENCE OF OKINAWAN KARATE-DO
by Shoshin Nagamine

"Nagamine's book will awaken in all who read it a new understanding of the Okinawan open-handed martial art."
—Gordon Warner
Kendo 7th dan, renshi

ESSENTIAL SHORINJIRYU KARATEDO
by Masayuki Kukan Hisataka

A well-rounded guide to this highly innovative and effective martial art. Describing preset forms, fighting combinations, and weapons, it is an excellent introduction to this comprehensive fighting system.

FILIPINO MARTIAL ARTS: CABALES SERRADA ESCRIMA *by Mark V. Wiley*

An excellent introduction to this deadly but graceful Filipino art of armed and unarmed combat. Packed full of information on the techniques, tactics, philosophy, spirituality, and history of the Filipino martial arts, this book is a vital addition to any martial arts library.

THE HAND IS MY SWORD: A KARATE HANDBOOK
by Robert A. Trias

The history, the fundamentals, the basic techniques, and katas are brought to life by over 600 illustrations in this book, which teaches that to master others one must first master oneself.

HSING-I: CHINESE INTERNAL BOXING
by Robert W. Smith and Allen Pittman

A superb introduction to the Chinese art of Hsing-i that both beginners and advanced practitioners can use to probe deeply into the secrets of one of the most complete systems of self-defense yet developed.

JUDO FORMAL TECHNIQUES
by Tadao Otaki and Donn F. Draeger

A comprehensive manual on the basic formal techniques of Kodokan Judo, the *Randori no Kata*, which provide the fundamental training in throwing and grappling that is essential to effective Judo.

KARATE: THE ART OF "EMPTY-HAND" FIGHTING
by Hidetaka Nishiyama and Richard C. Brown

A highly acclaimed, unexcelled treatment of the techniques and principles of karate. Includes over 1,000 easy-to-follow illustrations and a thorough review of the history and organization of the art.

KARATE BREAKING TECHNIQUES *by Jack Hibbard*

The first book solely on the art and technique of breaking. Over 500 outstanding photographs show clearly how to execute breaks in a simple step-by step manner.

THE KARATE DOJO: TRADITIONS AND TALES OF A MARTIAL ART *by Peter Urban*

This book discusses in detail the *dojo*, or training hall. Gives anecdotes on the origins and history of karate, as well as on the important role it has played in history.

KARATE'S HISTORY AND TRADITIONS
by Bruce A. Haines

Written by a historian, this book both describes the origins of karate and explains the importance of Zen in the serious study of karate.

THE NINJA AND THEIR SECRET FIGHTING ART
by Stephen K. Hayes

The ninja were the elusive spies and assassins of feudal Japan. This book explains their lethal system of unarmed combat, unique weapons, and mysterious techniques of stealth.

NINJA WEAPONS: CHAIN AND SHURIKEN
by Charles V. Gruzanski

The only book on the Masaki-ryu, which uses the "ten-thousand power chain" and *Shuriken-jutsu*, which uses metal projectiles developed to help swordless ninja defeat armed samurai.

PA-KUA: EIGHT-TRIGRAM BOXING
by Robert W. Smith and Allen Pittman

This book outlines the history and philosophy of the martial art based on the Pa-kua, the eight trigrams of the I-Ching. A definitive guide to this internal Chinese martial art.

THE SECRETS OF JUDO: A TEXT FOR INSTRUCTORS AND STUDENTS
by Jiichi Watanabe and Lindy Avakian

A fully illustrated text on the major *waza*—includes the most important throws, strangles, and pins. An indispensable introduction to judo and its basics.

SECRETS OF SHAOLIN TEMPLE BOXING
edited by Robert W. Smith

Abundantly and attractively illustrated, this book presents the essence of Shaolin in three sections—its history, its fundamentals, and its techniques—gleaned from a rare Chinese text.

SECRETS OF THE SAMURAI
by Oscar Ratti and Adele Westbrook

"Ratti and Westbrook have captured the breadth and depth of feudal Japanese *bujutsu* and its modern progeny. Anyone with a genuine interest in the roots of Japanese military tradition and martial arts should have this book."
—*The Journal of Asian Martial Arts*

SHAOLIN: LOHAN KUNG FU
by P'ng Chye Khim and Donn F. Draeger

A clearly written manual giving detailed explanations of the special elements of South China's Lohan style of Shaolin, including the Lohan pattern in both solo and partner forms.

SHOTO-KAN KARATE: THE ULTIMATE IN SELF-DEFENSE *by Peter Ventresca*

The first few chapters of this valuable book are devoted to warming-up exercises, stances, blocking, and kicking techniques that prepare the student for the study and practice of two kata—*Bassai No. 1* and *Tekki No. 1.*

THE SPORT OF JUDO
by Kiyoshi Kobayashi and Harold E. Sharp

"This Kodokan-approved book answers the long-felt need for a good, practical introduction to judo, . . . splendidly illustrated." —*The New York Times*

TAE KWON DO: SECRETS OF KOREAN KARATE
by Sihak Henry Cho

This book teaches Tae Kwon Do, probably the strongest form of self-defense known. This Korean form of karate is highly competitive, and its practice is one of the best ways to achieve mental and physical fitness.

T'AI-CHI: THE "SUPREME ULTIMATE" EXERCISE
by Cheng Man-ch'ing and Robert W. Smith

Written by one of the leading Yang-style experts, who studied directly under the legendary Yang Cheng-fu (d. 1935), this book illustrates Cheng's famous short form and includes a translation of the *T'ai-Chi Ch'uan Classics*.

THIS IS KENDO *by Junzo Sasamori and Gordon Warner*

The first book in English to describe the origin and history of kendo, its basic principles and techniques, its etiquette, and its relation to Zen. A must for any serious martial artist.

THE WEAPONS AND FIGHTING ARTS OF INDO-NESIA *by Donn F. Draeger*

Discover the ancient and modern combative forms of the Indonesian archipelago. As varied as the islands themselves, the styles described in this classic work include mysterious and deadly unarmed and weapons arts.

WING CHUN KUNG-FU: VOLUMES 1, 2, and 3
by Dr. Joseph W. Smith

A comprehensive series on this highly effective Chinese martial art. Volume 1 covers the basic forms and principles; Volume 2 illustrates fighting and grappling; and Volume 3 shows weapons and advanced techniques.

ZEN SHAOLIN KARATE: THE COMPLETE PRAC-TICE, PHILOSOPHY & HISTORY *by Nathan Johnson*

The ultimate interpretation of karate forms. A book that breaks the barriers separating karate, kung fu, and aikido, it revolutionizes the way preset forms are applied in all karate styles.